Travel Safety Tips for Women

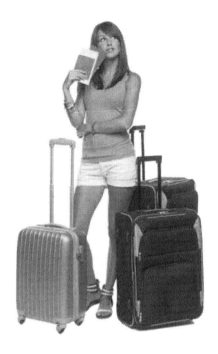

How to Travel Safely Around the Country or Around the World

Dueep Jyot Singh

Mendon Cottage Books

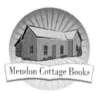

JD-Biz Publishing

All Rights Reserved.

No part of this publication may be reproduced in any form or by any means, including scanning, photocopying, or otherwise without prior written permission from JD-Biz Corp Copyright © 2015

All Images Licensed by Fotolia and 123RF.

Disclaimer

The information is this book is provided for informational purposes only. It is not intended to be used and medical advice or a substitute for proper medical treatment by a qualified health care provider. The information is believed to be accurate as presented based on research by the author.

The contents have not been evaluated by the U.S. Food and Drug Administration or any other Government or Health Organization and the contents in this book are not to be used to treat cure or prevent disease.

The author or publisher is not responsible for the use or safety of any diet, procedure or treatment mentioned in this book. The author or publisher is not responsible for errors or omissions that may exist.

Warning

The Book is for informational purposes only and before taking on any diet, treatment or medical procedure, it is recommended to consult with your primary health care provider.

Our books are available at

1. Amazon.com
2. Barnes and Noble
3. Itunes
4. Kobo
5. Smashwords
6. Google Play Books

Table of Contents

Going Solo 1
Travel Safety Tips for Women 1
    Introduction 4
    Getting Prepared to Travel 7
    Traveling Internationally 13
        When to Call Your Embassy for Help? 13

    Potential Trouble Situations 16
        Dress Code 17

    What to Have in Your Purse? 22
        Woman Safety App 22

    Money Money Money 26
    While on a Journey 30
    In an Unknown Neighborhood 33
    Parleying in the Local Lingo 36
    Harassment 43
        Harassed by Flirts 48

    Silence is Golden 50
    Meeting New Acquaintances 53
        Driving Rules 54

    Travel Plans 57
    Conclusion 59
    Author Bio 61
    Publisher 72

Introduction

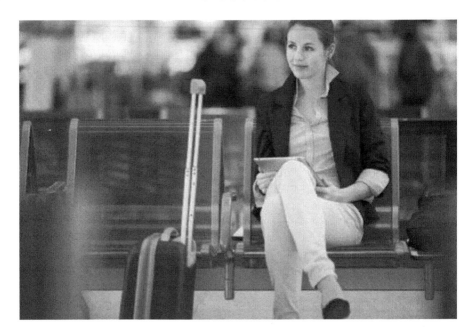

Going Solo...

Thanks to the world shrinking due to more advanced transport facilities, more and more women are taking the first step of traveling to other countries and exploring the new cultures, and horizons open to them.

It is the first step outside your own safe and secure circle, which is rather daunting. So for most of us Going solo is not something which people normally do because let me tell you frankly, I have noticed that a number of my women friends, colleagues and acquaintances consider any sort of traveled to be a bore.

Who really wants to undergo the hassle of being a woman all lonesome on her own traveling to a strange country or city? Traveling all alone in your own country or abroad, – you must be joking, DJ.

This attitude was rather surprising, because I took travelling alone to be a part and parcel of my own lifestyle, while growing up and I definitely did not have any hassle in picking up my small travelling bag and catching my train, all alone on a long journey, even when I was 15.

But then I was just going from one known destination to another known destination. So I did not bother much about the safety aspects, then, because I knew both destinations well.

So for me, at that time, Going solo was the rule, and not an exception.

But things changed later, while working. It was a different matter altogether. I never knew when the call would come from the top for me to get myself to such and such place by such and such time to attend such and such a meeting or meet XYZ.

At that time, I always had a bag packed in a corner because I never knew when I had to drop everything and fly down to all corners of the compass on official duty.

Sometimes I had my team of colleagues and juniors with me. Sometimes I was needed to go alone. And half of them just hated the idea of traveling because they were not used to it. Even when tickets, hotel stay, transport and all other facilities were laid out for them, they just did not want to go and see a brand-new place and experience a brand-new culture. How much they have missed out of life.

This book is for all those adventurous souls who want to go out somewhere and experience new experiences, but there always daunted by the thought that it is not safe for women to travel anywhere in their own country or outside. And definitely not traveling solo in this world full of crime, and xenophobia.

This book is to explode some of those myths. This book is also going to give you lots of useful information about safety tips for women traveling alone, based on my experiences, as well as the experiences of my other peripatetic friends. Also, there are some amusing anecdotes and episodes recounted to me by my well-traveled father, which may not exactly touch on safety, but can touch on some of the experiences that you may face when visiting a new country!

So let the adventure begin.

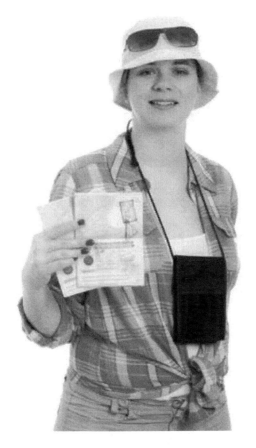

Have passport will travel!

Getting Prepared to Travel

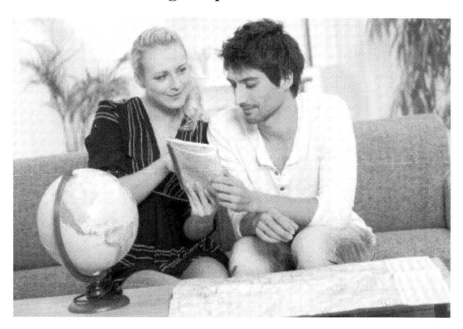

That's where I am going!

If you have never traveled outside your own city – and you will be surprised to see that a large majority of us come in that category – you may find it rather traumatic to have to travel to another place. Especially when you know nothing about that place.

In your 20s and 30s, it would have been rather adventurous for you to move to a new setting or location. That is the natural, inborn wandering instinct of a human being, looking for another place to settle where he can feel safe and his family can be protected.

That was the state of mind and society millenniums ago. But today we are fortunate that most of us can afford to travel, just to enjoy a holiday and come back to our own safe surroundings. But if you are a first-time traveler, be tranquil.

You are now going to launch on a new adventure. You are going to a place, which either you know, or which you do not know.

The safety rules and regulations for both destinations are going to be different.

If you are going to a place you know, and you are staying there with relatives, you do not have to worry much about really strict and stringent safety aspects, because after all it is your own little neck of the woods. You know the nearest police station.

You also know that you have relatives to take care of you in case you meet with an accident. You just have to board your flight, and your relatives will be there to pick you up at your destination.

But what if you are going to a place for the first time? What if you have never been abroad before? You have heard such terrible tales about the safety aspect of traveling in a place you need to visit. Should you ask your boss to send somebody else? Or do you want to take the chance of the adventure of a lifetime and go yourself?

That is when you need lots of mental and emotional preparation to take the first giant step into one can almost say a brand-new world.

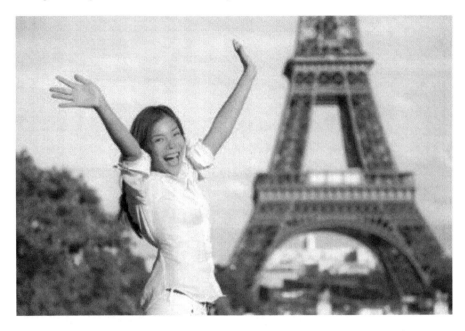

I am really here, at last!

So you begin with extensive preparation beforehand. Common sense is what you are going to need here, and these tips are such practical tips, which you can use in a matter of fact, and sensible manner right away.

First point is – how long are you going to be away? If it is just a trip for a week, or less, do not take more than one small bag. Traveling light is the first rule. Do not make your bag so heavy that it is impossible for you to pick it up and run in case of an emergency.

Let me give you one example. I was not traveling solo at that time, but with my father and brother on the road from Srinagar – Kashmir – to Ladakh in '86. Our tickets back home had been booked from Leh, and we had to get there in the next five days.

And all the traffic had stopped between these two cities because of landslides… So if my father had not been adventurous, we would still be sitting in Srinagar and wringing our hands helplessly. Instead he just asked one of the truck drivers to point us towards the general direction of Leh and we started to walk! 416 km on the most hazardous, unknown and perilous road known in the Indian subcontinent.

We had one sleeping bag each, a backpack full of food, a bottle full of water, and one small bag with just our clothes and toiletry items. And *nothing extra*. And we were launching on a new adventure through unknown land.

My father must have been terrified because he had the responsibility of his two teenage children on his hands, one of them a girl. But he never let it show as we marched down the road loudly singing and swinging to *make-believe you are in a jungle movie, watch the baby elephants go by, the beat is groovy…*[1]

---

[1] https://www.youtube.com/watch?v=t3HrNyoRylQ - Film Hatari! And our most preferred marching song. Our next noisy choice was Gee ma I wanna go home, only I and my brother sang "Colonel, we wanna go home". And we did!

Enjoy the lyrics –
http://lyricsplayground.com/alpha/songs/g/geemaiwannagohome.shtml

And so we put our faith and fate in the hands of God, and started to walk towards them thar hills, yonder.

However, 2 miles ahead, we found an Army supply convoy, which was the only transport available and they were kind enough to take us to their next base. And so we got to our destination a day before D-Day, on any transport available, truck and Army convoys, trucks, walking, etc. And we reached there only to find that the flight back had been canceled, due to bad weather!

When I analyze the safety aspect of such a hazardous venture, I marvel at the total innocence of three voyagers going through unknown lands, with just one map and a will to reach our destinations. But somehow we never found the idea of fear touching us, because we had been brought up that way.

Most of us are not fortunate enough to have that sort of wild and woolly[2] upbringing. That is why they would have stayed at Srinagar and many sensible people would have done that. So do not go off traipsing into the wild, like we did, but if you have to, make sure that you have packed light.

---

[2] You have my permission to say woolly headed.

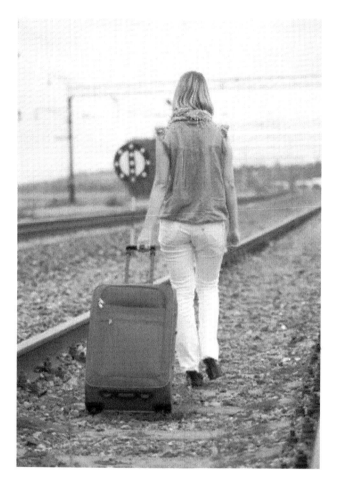

I was talking about the wilderness. Let us talk about the even more dangerous concrete jungle.

Start by getting to know all about the city you are going to visit. There are going to be some areas which you are definitely not going to explore. That is because even sensible people in the city keep away from those areas because of law and order problems. You are definitely not the Amazon queen Hippolyta. So keep away from that area.

Many women who get mugged in strange cities should know that they are **not** going to get any help from the local police, because after all, they were *asking for it,* exploring the tough localities at night, just for fun. "Asking for it" unfortunately is the catchword, which is being used globally by authorities in order to cover up their own lethargic attitude towards any untoward incident.

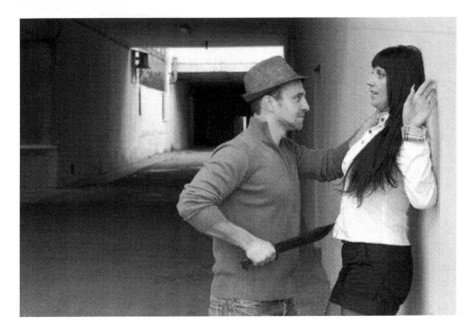

This woman comes under the category of just asking to become a statistic. Keep to well-populated places.

In many parts of the world, even today, a tourist – man or woman who has been mugged or even assaulted cannot be sure that the perpetrators would we bought to justice ever. Often this incident is going to be hushed up by the authorities or you may be asked not to take on the extra tension of a police case. This tension naturally means police inquiries, and other publicity, especially if the local news channels get to know all about any untoward incident in relation to a woman tourist.

These channels have absolutely no intention of helping you get justice. They are interested in their TRP ratings. And so your plight is going to be broadcast all over the world and you are going to be left with traumatic memories. Naturally, why would you want to visit that country again?

All this could have been avoided if you had had the good sense to stay in your safe room at night and not go exploring the nightclubs in some particular notorious area just to show how bold and brave you were.

Traveling Internationally

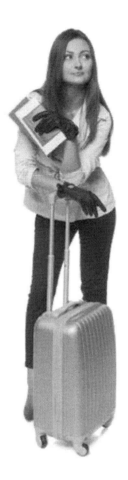

When to Call Your Embassy for Help?

Being a foreigner in a foreign land alas means often even more prejudice or I can say down right callousness on the part of authorities in matters of law and order.

So if you are in a foreign country and find yourself in the soup, the only source of help is going to be your country's consulate or the Embassy. Even then, possibly they are going to say that they are helpless under some particular circumstances, because "you know what this country is and why did you follow its rules?"

So that means that you should not go to a foreign country, without knowing the country's strict rules and regulations, hoping that you are going to be protected by your Embassy, if you happen to get into trouble.

For example, if you find yourself caught with drugs in many countries in Southeast Asia, – especially Thailand – and many parts of the Middle East, you are definitely going to find yourself shut up in Klink and $_{the}$ key thrown away without any chance of a plea bargain. No loud talking about you being the citizen of some particular Western or Eastern country is going to save you and your Embassy personnel are going to be the first to tell you that.

So when can they really help you?

Well, when I was visiting Egypt, I found my pocket picked. My plane tickets were gone, along with my passport, my money and here I was up the proverbial creek without a paddle. That was because I had been stupid enough to carry my passport and tickets with me, for some last-minute shopping.

The local police looked at me and said that it would take about three weeks for them to get any sort of results pertaining to my lost documents and money, and I had to leave the next day! And then, I had to pay my hotel bill for my stay, before I could check out.

So what did I do? I had already made sure that I had enough of money in my account back home to meet such a contingency. So make sure that you have lots of money in your account, back at home to pay for your tickets, and your hotel charges.

Our Embassy there was helpful in that they made duplicate travel documents, because I had the Photostats of my passport, my identity card, my visa page, and my plane tickets to show them. These had been left in the hotel room.

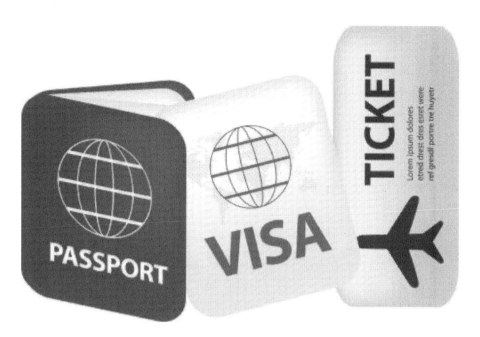

Make copies of these documents. Leave one set with relatives or family at home.

But somehow, those officials were rather wary about lending me hard cash with which to pay my hotel bill and other dues. I do not blame them for that because I know that every foreign Embassy in every country is faced with hard luck stories from tourists and a large percentage of them are Cons. So , in such cases, they are justifiably once bitten, twice shy.

So make Photostat copies of all your important documents and place them carefully in a separate bag. This bag is going to be kept in your hotel room safe, along with 60% of your money. That means even if your today's budget is picked when you were out exploring the markets, you know that you have enough of funds to help you get back.

Potential Trouble Situations

Do not drink alcoholic beverages when you are traveling solo. This is something many women would not have done, 20 years ago, but then at that time they would also not have been traveling alone.

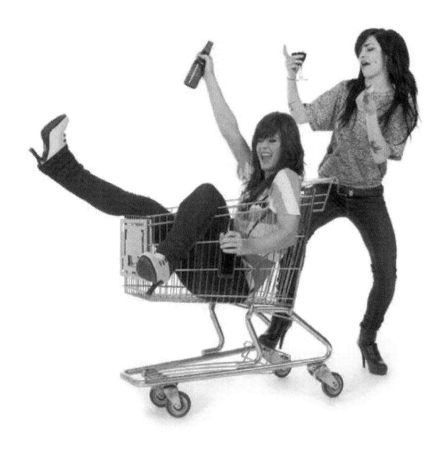

Being a party girl in your own town may be acceptable, but do not make a fool of yourself in a strange city.

But the brave brash new generation which is more adventurous would not find it strange to walk into any pub and down a number of snifters, just because she is feeling lonely or lonesome tonight.

This is "asking for it" in no uncertain terms. You may find yourself assaulted and molested, because let us face it, when anybody wants to molest you, he is going to justify this action with she was acting so... well, let us say, available, how did I know that she was not that sort?

Also, if you are traveling in the Middle East or in any other country where you know the mindset of the male population is that of the dark ages – women should be docile, and kept in their place – do not provoke any sort of action or confrontation by showing that you are a 21st-century broad-minded liberated and emancipated female.

Unfortunately, the mindset of many of the people in many parts of the world is that women from the West do not mind attention, sometimes even forcibly, because they are used to it. Naturally, this attitude is there a way of justifying molesting a foreign tourist all on her own. Sadly, such incidents are growing in number in Southeast Asia, and on the Indian subcontinent.

So if you are traveling alone here, it is your job to protect yourself. What is considered normal behavior on the streets of Paris or in New York is going to horrify the onlookers in more conservative countries. That includes public displays of affection.

Dress Code

This is also where we come to dress. I have traveled all over with just three changes of underclothing, two pairs of jeans, and two shirts in a small bag. This is of course apart from the traveling gear, which I am going to wear while traveling. This gear is going to be a loose fitting shirt and baggy trousers with a long scarf when traveling in India or in other conservative countries like Malaysia, Burma, Thailand, etc.

Leave your shorts and skimpy figure hugging T-shirts at home.

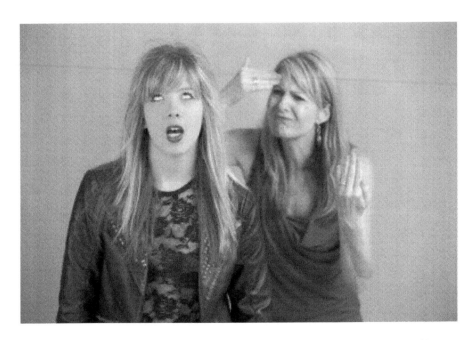

What is wrong with you, do you mean to go off on a trip, dressed like that?

The parent has a reason to be scared and terrified. The teenager is absolutely no inkling of what could happen to her. Instead she is under the impression that mom is creating, in her usual way. Most of us are incapable of listening to good sense, because we are so used to doing anything opposite to what our well-wishers tell us to do.

If this girl goes on a trip all alone, and dressed like that, she is soon going to be part of that city's law and order statistics.

Your traveling outfit should be comfortable enough for you to be able to sleep in it. It should also be rough and tough, which means that it should be able to bear rough weather, spills, stains, dust and other travel related activities.[3].

---

[3] https://www.youtube.com/watch?v=-jSMUI3L2EY

So when you are exploring, what do you need to have in a traveling pouch wrapped around your waist? Leave your passport in your hotel safe – if you think it is not safe in your room – and have a photocopy of your identity, person to contact in an emergency, your own identification, and any other relevant documents in one part of the money bag/traveling pouch/belt.

You can buy these belts anywhere in your city at reasonable prices. Make sure your belt is sturdy and wraps around your waist snugly. Once it is on, you are just going to wear your shirt over it. Do not wear it outside your shirt as a hip belt. Someone may just slash it with a sharp blade, and you may never know where it has fallen.

See the clothes Kangy Ranaut wears in this clip of "Queen", while travelling and exploring new cities. Get Kurtas like that, which are comfortable and appropriate to the weather.

This is an escapist movie, so I would not advise you to go drinking and dancing at night, in discos in Paris. You may find someone there Asking You to Prove It!

Kurtas are unisex rough and tough cotton shirts. You can see what they look like on this URL

http://www.ebay.com/sch/i.html?_from=R40&_trksid=p2050601.m570.l1131 3.TR0.TRC0.H0.Xwoman+Kurtas.TRS0&_nkw=woman+Kurtas&_sacat=0

They are available universally, so if you find them in your city and at a reasonable price, get some your own size!

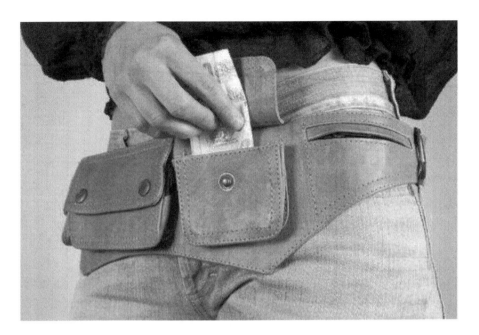

Her shirt should be long enough to cover the belt, after she has put our money in it. That is why spoke about loose fitting kurtas!

Do not travel around in a city with a hand purse, which occupies one hand. Have a shoulder length bag which you are going to sling crosswise across the length of your body.

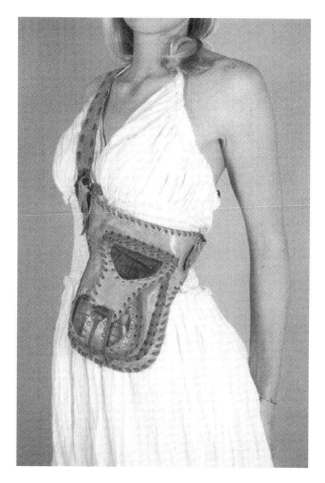

Best position for your bag while traveling – in front, and not behind you, or swinging on your hip.

Do not sling it over one shoulder, because that is going to make it very easy for someone to try and grab it. As for a hand purse, the handles are so flimsy that the moment somebody grabs it, you find yourself clutching the handles – even if it is an expensive Hermes or any other expensive brand-name, made wholesale in Hong Kong or in mainland China – and there is your purse gone with the wind.

What to Have in Your Purse?

Your purse should have a guidebook, a city map and a well charged cell phone, lots of paper and a number of ball pens. Do not overfill your purse with extra toiletry goods which may come into your way, if you need to get to your cell phone in an emergency.

Some people go traveling around with their cell phones clutched in their hands. Here they are with one hand occupied. Just imagine someone tries to grab your purse. What I you going to do with just one hand? So have your cell phone at an easily accessible place.

Woman Safety App

I do not know about safety apps for women in the USA or in other countries, but in India the Udaipur police launched a woman safety app called Pukar ["Call"] in December, 2014.

You can learn more about it on Google play on your cell phone.

https://play.google.com/store/apps/details?id=com.pukar&hl=en

It is still in the testing stage, but I think the idea is very revolutionary.

If it is left to me, I would give the makers of the safety application, the best and most sensible creativity award for 2014. You do not need a Wi-Fi connection to launch it. This is the reason why I want to recommend it for top prize for most useful application for women safety. With this, you can connect to two – three of your loved ones and the nearest police station immediately, in times of danger.

I believe there is soon going to come a time when every woman traveling outside her own city is going to have her own country's version of Pukar downloaded on her cell phone or smartphone.

I do not know about the money charged by international talk time providers for your cell phone, because I am talking about the cell phone charges in my country. We have different rates for local charges and different rates for outstation charges which come under the roaming category.

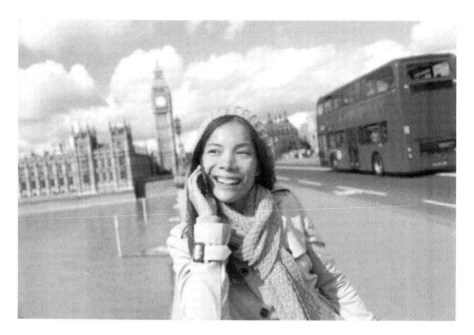

I remember going for my annual holiday to my brother's place last year, and he wanted to borrow my smart phone.

He made a grimace when he saw my talk time, which was somewhere around USD50. He immediately recharged it to USD500. His reasoning was so logical, but so many of us do not think of it.

We are on "roaming" or "international charges" when we go to a strange city, if we have not bought a local phone or SIM card. The phone charges are going to be more than the local charges you paid in your city.

So now let us imagine that you are in Denver and you are trying to contact your relatives in, let us say, Birmingham.

You have no international dial landline phone around you. You have to rely on your cell phone. And suddenly it starts to beep that your talk time is over and you have not even managed to shout for help or to give them relevant information. So here you are with this expensive piece of junk, which needs to be charged again with talk time.

There are service providers which allow you to recharge immediately and continue talking, but just imagine you are stranded in a not so safe area. Are you going to stand there recharging your cell phone or look for the nearest police station?

And if your battery decides to say goodbye at that particular moment, because it has not been charged, well, it is all your fault, and I definitely do not have any sympathy for such criminal carelessness.

Why blame it when it is your own entire fault for not charging it?

So why am I being so needlessly harsh about this point, you may ask? Well, that is because I have experienced this bit of stupidity myself. One fine morning I grabbed my smart phone on the way to the office and that was the day my scooter decided to skid on the wet road, efficiently trapping my leg underneath it.

So when I took out my cell phone to contact my office and my family that I was all right, alive and kicking on one leg, my smart phone beeped, and said "connect your charger". And before I could dial any number, the battery went dead.

Luckily, the traffic police had their own communication systems ready at hand to reassure office and family. But how helpless I felt with this expensive piece of sophisticated machinery which did not come to my aid, just because of my own carelessness.

 Have a smart phone, which is reliable and has a long battery time. Also look at other tracking aids which can help keep you safe.

This is where GPS comes in. Make sure that you have GPS tracking on your cell phone. At least your last known position is going to be known. And then if you disappear, there is going to be some blip going beep beep beep to tell the authorities looking for you where they can find you or where they can find your cell phone.

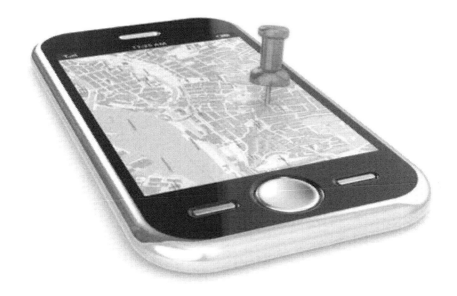

That is where she is!

Money Money Money

Call me paranoid, but I never keep my money in just one place when I am traveling. I never wear jewelry. Leave your diamonds and gold at home. You are not going there for a fashion show, unless of course you are going there for a fashion show, which means that you are going to be escorted everywhere, and your safety is the responsibility of your sponsors!

Do not show off about how rich you are, or tell stories about your bulging bank account. It is a known fact that even today, women are kidnapped in many parts of the world and held to ransom, because they boasted a bit about their rich rich families. So if you have a tendency of exaggerating your financial status, learn to keep your mouth shut in public.

If you are traveling abroad, keep just one credit card and do not bring lots of cash. Use travelers checks and just a small amount of cash.

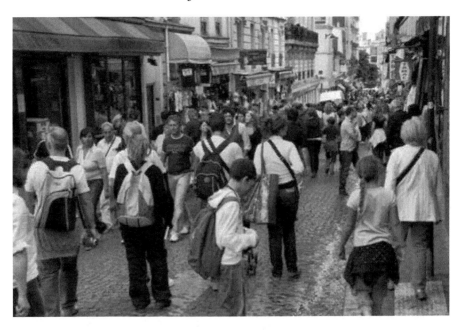

Shopping in the city you are visiting is an exhilarating experience, as long as you know, and have limited the amount of money that you intend to spend on items brought from here.

So how much money do you carry around with you when you are exploring the city? I never put all my eggs in one basket. I have money in three places, when I am out exploring a city, and also in three places, during the journey from one place to another.

One place is the purse, which I am going to open when I am shopping. It is not going to be full of notes flashing and tempting pickpockets. My demeanor is that "I am not a tourist. I know how to shop in this city." That means I know all about the local currency and its equivalent in the money of my own country. I also know that when I am shopping the prices are going to being inflated specially for me.

Bargaining can only be done if you know the lingo and the culture. I remember a Reader's Digest joke of the 60s, about a lady visiting Italy, and having a really good time bargaining for three hours for some items. She managed to get the price reduced to $1/8^{th}$ the original price, and before payment, she said "now that I am paying you for these three items, you may want to add that small vase to the packet, free. " And the shop keeper smiled widely and said, "oh no, for you signora, we do something else and better. We start bargaining again!"

So if you have the time to bargain, do so. But do not let the people in the shop know that your purse is full of hard-earned dollars.

That means you need to have limited money, which is easily accessible in your purse. Stick to that budget when you are shopping, and the moment it is finished, come back home.

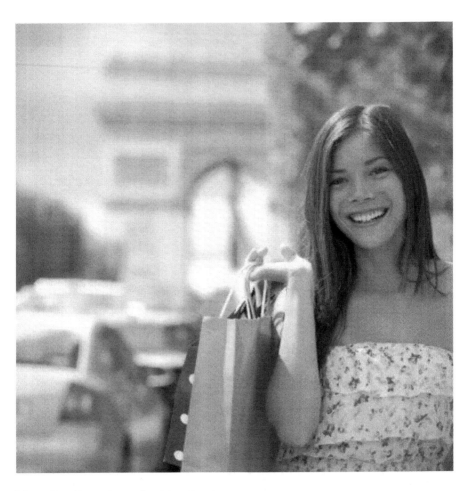

Now that I am here, just try to stop me...

But what if you find something which is a bargain? That is when you are going to be needing the extra money in your second pocket, which you have secured with a safety pin. If you want access to it, go to the nearest retiring room and take it out of your secret pocket.

Make sure nobody sees you doing that! Because there may be a chance that casual witnesses may go talking to their acquaintances about that tourista with money hidden underneath her shirt, and there you are, a potential future mugging statistic.

I normally put my third cash reserve, in my flying boots when I traveled in jeans, T-shirt and knee length boots, in the days of my peripatetic youth and up to my 30s.

By God's grace, I never needed to ever have access to that money, which was enough to get me home, back to my original destination city, in case of an emergency. Being a proper little tough, I also had an army knife in its sheath given to me by my grandfather to protect myself. Of course I never used it or had occasion to, thankfully, but somehow its mere presence made me feel more secure!

This was in the 80s and 90s. I switched to Kurta pajama (loose trousers with an elastic band) in the 2000s, with plenty of pockets. So have these pockets sewn in your shirts.

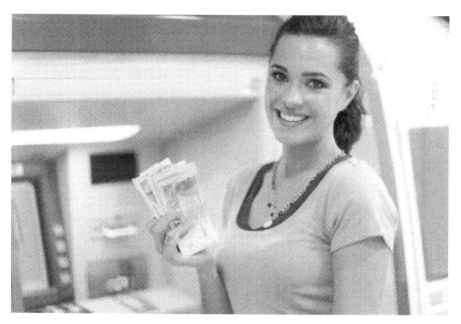

Do not use your ATM card in the cash slot at night. If you need to withdraw cash, do it in a busy place, in the day.

While on a Journey

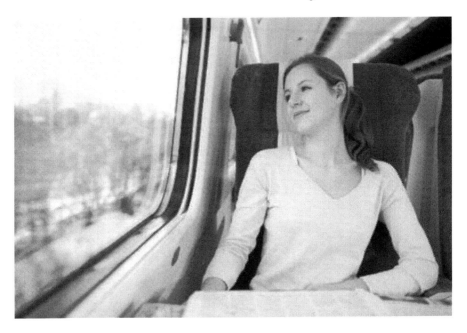

If you are leaving a new city for another new destination, visit the bus stop or the train station the day before you have to leave. Find out how to get there. How long does it take to reach that place from your hotel? How long is your journey going to take?

Confirm the departure time. If your flight is late at night and you have booked out from your hotel to reach the airport in time, you are safe in the lounge. But if somehow you manage to book out before time and have time hanging on your hands, do not decide to go shopping. Get into a café near the airport or an Internet café. You are going to be safe there. Also, you can spend your time sending mails to your near and dear ones that you are on your way back.

If you are in an empty compartment, avoid sleeping in it, unless it is of course in a country where you have First-Class/AC accommodation and you can lock it from inside. Also, in many parts of Asia, the railways have ladies compartments, where no man may enter. In fact, they may ask you if you want your ticket in a ladies compartment when you are booking it in these countries.

Abroad, if you are in an empty compartment, you may want to change your seat for another one where you have a family around you. It is going to cost you a little bit extra. Abroad, we have couchettes, for overnight journeys where other like-minded tourists can rest safely. These can be locked and they are often monitored by attendants. You are going to wake up safe and rested with all your belongings safe and sound.

If you are traveling in Spain or in France, you can ask for compartments with women roommates in overnight trains, especially when it is not the tourist season. In France, the conductor's room has a one compartment, which is set aside for women passengers, but it is very expensive. So it is better to ask for all the options in the country in which you are traveling and ask to bunk with other women tourists and passengers. If you are lucky, you are going to get them. But do not count on it!

So, how safe are you in a ladies compartment? You may say that things happen to me, but having traveled such a lot, there is a chance that I may come up against some bad apples, even in my fellow passengers.

I was traveling on a long trip, in a ladies compartment, where I found out that my fellow passenger had to get off at her destination somewhere at midnight. I am rather a light sleeper, and besides, I do not sleep too well when I am on a journey.

10 minutes before we had to reach her destination and I was supposedly asleep, I felt a sort of tug at the chain under my seat. I had chained my suitcase when I had entered the compartment and she did not know it. She had not seen the chain, and she had decided that a little bit of petty larceny would not come amiss, as she was reaching her destination in a couple of minutes.

I just opened one eye and hooted sleepily, "hey, "auntie", it is chained. So do not bother yourself. Bye."

She did not say bye and I went off to sleep serenely.

So take things like this as adventures and par for the course. That means chaining your suitcase or baggage to your own seat, in such a manner that any sort of tug on it will have you waking up and saying, do not bother yourself.

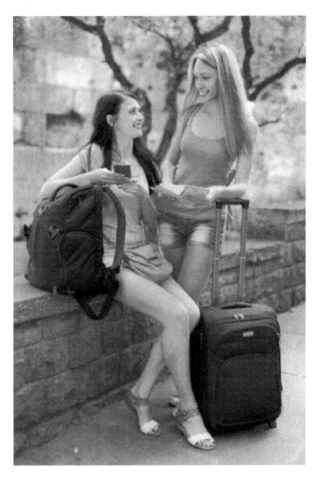

In an Unknown Neighborhood

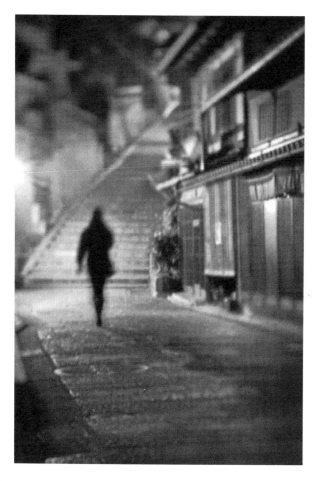

So not safe or sensible.

When you are walking in an unfamiliar neighborhood, act like you know where you are going. It is better if you do a little bit of research on how to get there beforehand.

You may also want to ask directions, sometimes. Ask a woman or ask people of a family, asking your question to the woman in the family. If you cannot see any woman around, go into the nearest store and asked for directions.

So do you talk to the local people or not? That depends, in the city and country in which you are. If you are traveling in Southeast Asia, you can talk to people, if you want to, but do not become over familiar.

Same goes for many countries in Europe. In the Middle East and in some Mediterranean countries like Syria, Jordan, Lebanon, etc. never ever talk to a man, on his own, as far as possible.

When I went visiting Rajasthan – in 2001, I was visiting a place I had not been to before. But I knew the country's language well, even though I could not speak the local dialect. I knew the people.

I also knew that I had relatives who had been living there for the last 30 years, so I could be a bit more adventurous.

So I found out all about the places where I could catch the cheapest transport. I also knew how to get to major city points like Swaasti gate. And then I walked to the Fort, from there through alleyways which are known only to the people of Jodhpur. Now this is something which I would not advise you to do in a strange city.

But the people there could see that even though I was a tourist[4], I had the self-confidence and purpose to know where I was going. Besides, I was following people going up to the Fort from the city. And this was in broad daylight. The area was well populated. And they could see from my face that any sort of attempt at harassment would bring about immediate retaliation, because my demeanor was definitely not flirty but grim.

Times have changed since then, and for the worse. Today I would not dare go through those areas alone, even though Jodhpur is very law-abiding. One can say that age has brought with it more common sense and discretion.

---

[4] My mistake. I was dressed in my exploring and traveling garb of black jeans, black polo neck shirt, black regimental cap with the legend "Outrams" embroidered on it and flying boots – with extra money and knife in the boots. And the costume of the region was Kurta , pajama and long scarf for well brought up women folk.

Besides, I often stopped at roadside shops and in a very polite voice asked the people there whether this was the way to the Fort? They asked me if I was a tourist and I told them that I had come visiting my relatives who had been staying here since the 50s, and this was my first visit, and this was such a beautiful place, all in the local lingo. This was very well appreciated.

And they told me other places to visit, including the palace. So there are nice people everywhere, and be nice to them, they are going to be nice to you. Remember that you are a visitor in their land. Let them have good memories of you.

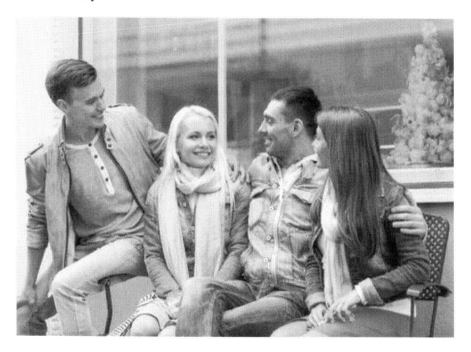

Making new friends in a strange city can be a memorable experience.

Parleying in the Local Lingo

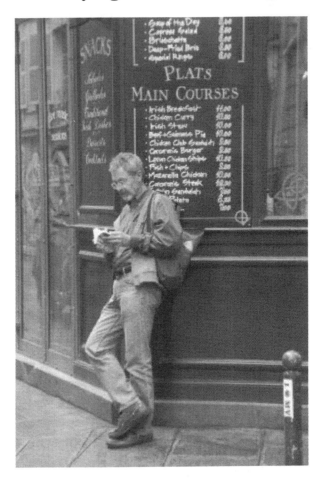

So what does my phrasebook say?

So now we come to another point. You should know the local lingo. It is no fun going to Düsseldorf, or to Paris, if you do not know a smattering of the language. At least you need to know enough to get yourself understood.

English is universal, but while traveling in India or in other Asian countries, you should know at least three regional languages and if you know somebody local, learn the local language from them along with the slang! That often comes very helpful.

I had learned a very polite statement of showing respect to my elders in the Rajasthani dialect from my aunt and I managed to trot it out loud, while I was talking to them in Hindi, and an elder joined in. He immediately voted me a very well brought up "girl child" even if I was in modern jeans and Man's shirt, which he would not allow his own womenfolk to wear, ever!

This reminds me about gestures and knowing the local language. When dad went visiting Paris in the 60s, he did not know even the basic ABC of French! He could not read it, he would not speak it. But he had gone off to see France without even a phrasebook, just for adventure's sake.

So he kept trying to ask his way to St. Michael, in Paris, and everybody giving him funny looks. They could not understand the English way he was pronouncing it.

Until a good soul had the patience to stand before this young man, saying St. Michael and gesturing with his hands with the universal gesture of where? So that is how dad managed to get to Sawn Mee shell!

This is the reason why he decided that his future children needed to be well-versed in all the important languages of the world, including French, because you never knew when you needed to speak them.

Also, his peripatetic job helped us speak languages and dialects up really fast, and naturally the first words we learned were cuss words and gutter slang. And though we very rarely used them as children, they often helped us when we grew up and had begun our own round of traveling around the globe.

I have managed to get my choice of wine...So how do I order what he is eating?

Talking about global gestures. So here is this hungry young man sitting in a Paris restaurant and wanting his lunch. Dad appreciates the fact that the waiter was very polite and his smile was more indulgent than patronizing, superior or contemptuous, when dad picked up the menu, looked at the prices and pointed to the dishes, without knowing what they were!

After that, he pointed to the breadsticks on the table, made a gesture of dipping them in a soup, and eating them. He was immediately brought a delicious lunch, along with a rich and enjoyable soup, which not only filled up his tummy, but was affordable.

He did the same thing in Italy. He did not know the language, but managed to get himself well understood with gestures. He remembers a young, bright eyed, good-looking Roman bambino waiting for him to throw a coin into the Fontana de Trevi in Rome, because he recognized him as a tourist from abroad, and possibly this tourist would have thrown in a coin of his own country! Excellent for his coin collection, bambino thought, as he dove in the water and grabbed the coin.

Dad had managed to order a glass beaker full of wine, in a nearby trattoria, just by pointing to it, and he had to reward such enterprise. So the boy got a gelato from dad as reward! Both of them did not know each other's language, but for that moment, adult and child, they had been bound by the silken thread of happy friendship and understanding.

So remember that the world is out there with magical miracle moments which you need to make, so when you are on holiday, make these moments yourself.

Why did not dad use phrase books you may ask? Believe it or not, the phrase books at that time still had English phrases like "the postilion has been struck by lightning!" So he used his own creativity to get himself understood.

Well, I guess I pronounced it right. He seems to have understood what I meant to say.

So here we come to the phrasebooks.

A Japanese tourist, visiting England for the first time happened to ask an Englishman, a phrase which he has learned from his English, Japanese phrasebook. So this is what he said, "What is time?"

The Englishman looked at him for a few seconds and then said pensively, "sorry, my friend, this is a question wise men have been asking themselves for thousands of years and I cannot really explain it to you."

In the same manner, a tourist feeling hungry, wanted to find a eating space in the vicinity. So he took out his phrasebook and looked for this phrase. "I want to eat." He tried it on a well-dressed man passing by, and the man put his hand in his pocket, took out five cents and gave it to him.

So those were the phrase books of yore!

Modern-day phrasebook publications are extremely useful. Besides, they have the sentence written out phonetically so that you can pronounce them right.

So what if you find yourself in a country where you are not very fluent in the language? And you do not have anybody near to teach you the local language, nor do you have access to a phrasebook.

Well, you are a woman, act helpless in front of the nearest woman! I am astonished to see how that works, and so beautifully, even though I am around 6 feet and am built on warrior lines!

But I just have to look as if I am as dumb as a dodo, give some sheepish smiles, say I am so sorry but with plenty of gestures and sign language, and the mother's instinct of the woman immediately will rise up and she is going to look after you!

Learn how to say "thank you so much, you are so kind, You have helped me," in the local language. Also show your sincerity in your voice when you are talking to them.

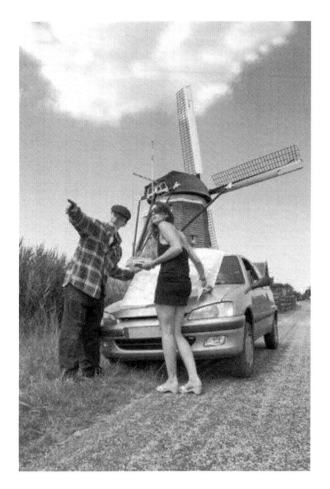

Never "demand" anything of anyone. The soft helpless look works even better than the aggressive "hey there, can you help me" attitude.

I learned this from my father. He has traveled to 30 countries, and even though he is not a woman, he knows everything about safety rules as well as other tips and techniques in order to facilitate your stay with the least amount of discomfort to you. For this you need a little bit of imagination and a little bit of showmanship.

In fact, even when he was around 70, he used to go off to pilgrimages in the mountains, in India, put off his garb of Cosmopolitan sophistication and become one with the people around him, as to garb and language.

And he spoke softly and looked so lost that the women pilgrims who had come there with their families on pilgrimage would immediately "adopt" Babbaji whose children were cruel enough not to accompany him on such long, arduous journeys. But then one knew the children of today, so thoroughly and utterly selfish.

And they were so kind to him, because he was so gentle, quiet and so helpless! He definitely should not have been left loose on his own.

Talk about deceptive garb and camouflage!

The nicest thing about such chance made friends is that 90% of the time you find out that they are lifelong friends forever. That is because all over the world, there are genuinely sincere and helpful people, especially those in India.

He never took his children along on these journeys, because he said half of the fun of adventuring would be lost, because we would be fussing around him and bothering about his safety!

In Europe, especially in a small town, if you have to talk to a man, make sure that he is accompanied by a woman. Focus more on her. The man is then going to give you the information you need. The same thing goes in Asia.

When you are moving in a city, do not do anything or wear anything that can focus attention on you. Keep to a group, if you are visiting tourist spots. Mingle with them.

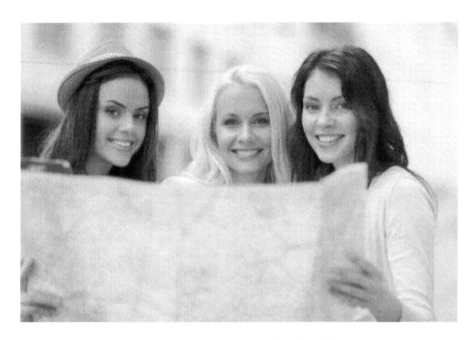

Find like-minded friends at your new destination, if you are going solo. It is good from the safety point of view, and you are also going to have company.

Harassment

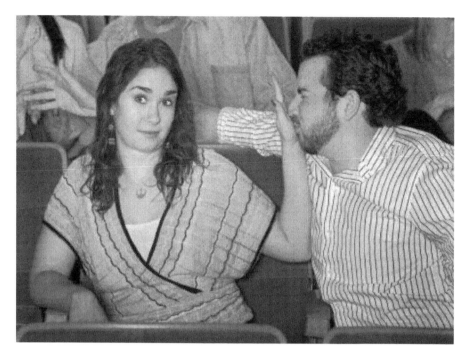

If you think you are being harassed, act firmly against it, right now.

The definition of harassment can encompass anything causing you overt mental and physical discomfort to clearly visible gestures and signs which you consider dangerous to your own well-being.

So what do you do if you are harassed? This is no time to be all ladylike and polite. Raise your voice. Use bad language in the local language. The worse the better. That is going to make people around you want to know why such a quiet sort of woman is using such filthy language.

You may want to bring their attention to the fact that the creature in front of you considers you to be a cheap tramp. You may also want to take out your cell phone and click his photo.

Passive behavior does not work when you are all alone. You have to be streetwise and overactive. Use aggressive body language, facial expressions and also learn how to say no in a very loud voice in the local language. This is when you are being crowded by someone trying to invade your own personal space. Keep repeating the no.

Is physical violence justified on your part? You being a woman are naturally geared not to be physically violent. You would rather curl up in a ball and hope that the unpleasantness is going to pass.

I am sorry to say, but that is the attitude which is being taken by a large number of us, because we are unable to face any sort of physical violence. So any aggressive attention from any man, and we are going to keep our mouths shut, because we have forgot about to shout, scream, yell, and use our hands and feet.

About a decade ago, there was a popular Bollywood blockbuster, starring one opinion's most talented and popular superstars – Nana Patekar. He has the power to make people think, in the story. During one scene, a timid and helpless woman keeps shouting for help as she is being kidnapped by pimps, to whom her sister-in-law had sold her.

He calmly tells her that God has given her a time to shout and to use her hands and feet to protect herself. He tells her son that that boy can protect his mother by stoning the kidnappers. Which, of course, the boy does. Shouting help, save me, someone save me would not bring a God down to the earth to save her. So she did and she saved herself. And then she picked up a stick and beat her sister-in-law as she so well deserved. Whistles from the audience, critic awards, superhit!

She acted and saved herself and thus got to know that she had the spirit to survive on her own. Otherwise, she would like any Barbara Cartland heroine have kept waiting for her hero, or for God to save her, instead of doing something constructive in that definitive moment.

So here is the SINGH self-protective formula that I apply, if I have ever need to protect myself in a situation where I found myself in personal jeopardy. That is the moment when you need to launch into action without your mind telling you that you may get hurt. The mind is geared to protect itself from physical hurt instinctively and naturally. So it is going to tell you not to do anything which can cause you physical hurt.

But this is one time when you need to override its dictates, and launch into action.

S for stomach – elbow or punch in it – I for instep – the upper portion of the foot, stamp on it, N for nose – the palm of the hand under the nose to break it –G- Knee in the groin region, and H- holler long and loud, for help or just yell bad words, or just about anything noisy. You are soon going to have an audience, to which you can shout for someone to call the police.

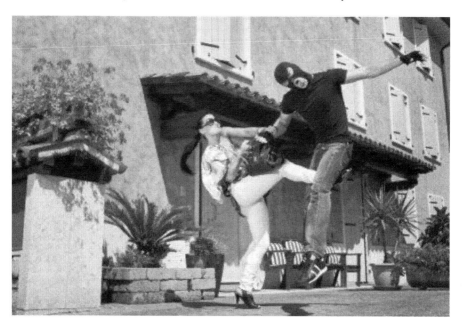

The G part of the self-defense instructions!

Someone will, unless all of them are zombies. In that case, you will have to continue this treatment until you can reach your cell phone and press your quick dial for the police.

Your cell phone quick dial should have the local police and your relatives phone numbers, as well as your local contacts numbers ready to access.

You may want to practice the quick dial, – do it ringing your own landline phone – because when things happen, they happen fast and practice is going to make you perfect.

Why do some women hate making a noisy fuss, especially when they are abroad, or when they are in a situation which is possibly going to put their own personal well-being in jeopardy?

Many of these women when questioned by the police replied that they were afraid to look foolish. What stupidity. It is your duty to look foolish and as noisily foolish as you can, because your instincts tell you that you are in danger. So Let the Tiger Roar.

If you are outside, you may want to start screaming and start pointing at the person who is following you. Or go into the nearest hotel and straight to the reception desk. Point that person out to the hotel staff. And then ask the hotel management to call you a cab or transport, which can take you to your own hostel or hotel.

Make sure that you know the name of your hotel, its contact number, how to get there, and address thoroughly before you go out exploring. Get their card and place it in your money purse.

Also, get the name of the contact person – hotel employee – in the hotel, to whom you have told your destination. Naturally, you are going to ask him/her beforehand on the easiest way to get there.

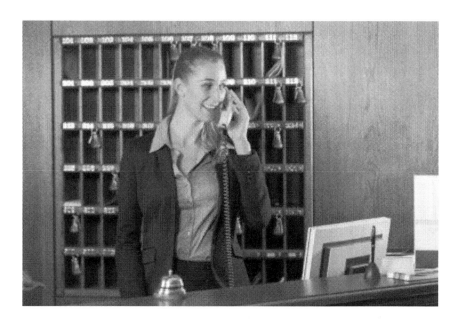

At least get to know one hotel employee, and have her phone number at hand.

Harassed by Flirts

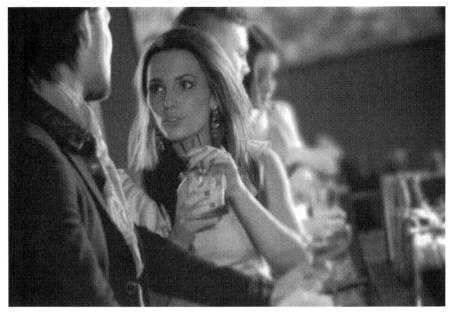

Just go away, will you? You are getting to be a pest.

That is all right, but he may not obey her. Because after all, she is alone at night, drinking in the bar.

If you find yourself being chatted up by some flirty guy who is out for a fling with a tourist, put on a wide smile and talk about your husband, your children and keep talking about your husband's interest in physical sports, especially boxing and karate.

Also tell him that you learned karate from your husband and is he interested in it? Do not give him the time to talk about himself. Keep blabbing about yourself. He is soon going to lose interest and go away. If you are in India, put on a fake wedding ring and a Mangal sutra. In any other country, you may want to put on the local symbol for a married woman.

I remember a friend like me, who also was a solo traveler. She used to visit a particular city very often, and stayed in one hotel where she became really friendly with an employee named Sandra. And as she was very pretty, she often found herself harassed by guys who would not take no for an answer.

One fine day, this persistent roadside Romeo decided that he did not really believe in the karate loving Marine who was resting in their room today and asked her to introduce him to her husband. My friend did not blink an eyelid. She saw that he was following her to her hotel, and hailed Sandra. "Sandy" she shouted, "is my husband feeling better?" the moment she entered the foyer.

"Of course ma'am, he was down there in the gym, boxing away, but he seems to be in a very bad temper. Do not you feel frightened when he is in such a mood?"

"Oh no," my friend said insouciantly, "I just introduce him to someone on whom he can take out his temper. Now this gentleman here has been trying to pick me up for the past half hour. He is going to enjoy talking to him! "And with a very wide smile, she beckoned roadside Romeo forward, who immediately decided that he had another appointment taking him far away from the irate and bad tempered Marine.

This story works best in Europe and in the USA. I am certain that there is going to be a roadside Romeo reading this [Remember the Mumbai terrorist attack when the exact minute by minute broadcast by the vulture like TV channels worked both ways in the dissemination of information to the terrorists and hindered the commando operations terribly.] He is immediately going to understand that this is an excuse, which can be used by a potential prospect. This is when you need the aid of a huge masculine presence.

Feminists are going to screech, but there are some times when an aggressive looking man is a very effective deterrent as well as visible security for a woman. So if any of your relatives, acquaintances and friends in the city which you are visiting is huge and hulking, do not hesitate in roping them in to protect the damsel in distress. But take permission from them first. They should not think that you are as needy as Twilight's Bella, and intent to cling on to them possessively after you leave the city. Men hate that sort of trapped feeling.

Silence is Golden

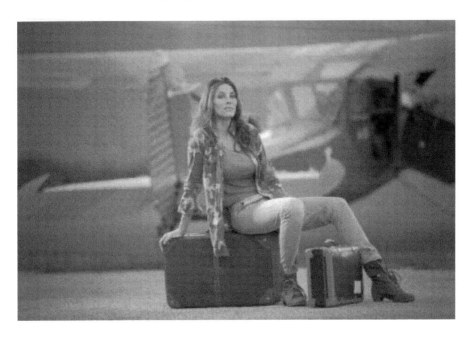

All packed and nowhere to go…

Never tell anyone that you are travelling all alone. Some people, especially in the East and Middle East want to know whether you are single or married.

Even if you are a spinster, do tell everyone that you are married and have been happily married for so many years, and keep talking about your children and your husband, and all about them.

Sometimes men use women to get to know all about other women who are possible potential targets. So lie unhesitatingly and use your own creativity. You may also want to show the inquisitive woman photos of your "family."

Be consistent in the story you are telling them. It is no use talking about your children Sean and Darrin and then calling them Sam and Derek three hours later. This is what happened with one of my rather scatterbrained friends, who remembered that the name started with S and with D and she could not really remember what they were.

So if you are talking about Sean and Derek, use their names a number of times, when you are recounting stories about them. At least then you will not forget them easily.

Unless, of course you come in the totally careless dim bulb category. Under such circumstances, you should not have been allowed to travel out alone without a keeper.

Talking about keepers, I remember one of my colleagues on a flight who got a bit carried away with her own imagination, to impress the opulent looking good looker on the seat next to her.

My seat was not next to hers, but I could hear and see her clearly.

To my great horror, the moment the plane took off, she started spinning a tale about her going all alone to the city, where, alas, she knew nobody. Her father? Oh, he was away somewhere, Tehran, or was it The Tyrol? She really could not keep track of all the names. And her mom? Well, she was somewhere in Australia with her third husband. She just hated being alone.

I could almost see Wolf licking his chops. So when we reached our destination, he stuck around, wanting to ask if he could escort her somewhere. His first setback was when he saw me coming out of the plane, and saying, "all right, Jenny, ready to go?" Jenny? This lady had told him that her name was Susan, you can call me Sue, giggle.

His second setback was when he saw our contacts coming to pick up our luggage and to welcome us. Hefty tough looking guys, all three of them.

He gave her a look of pitiful disappointment and nearly pouted. This beautiful lady had been pulling his leg throughout the journey, and to such an extent that he needed a pair of binoculars to see his toes.

And then she had the sheer effrontery to tell him how much she had enjoyed the journey, and she had been talking out of the hat, all the while, because she did not want to give him the opportunity to ask for her contact address and cell phone number.

Men had this bad tendency of doing that whenever she found herself traveling.

Now my friend "Sue" may have enjoyed herself very much, but she knew that we would not be alone at our final destination. If you are going alone somewhere, do not ever try out this stunt.

Hitch hiking at dusk or at night? That's a No, No, Nanette. Be sensible.

Meeting New Acquaintances

If you have been invited to meet someone, and he has chosen the rendezvous spot, make sure that it is a public place. Tell him that you are living with a number of roommates in a hostel with a curfew. Bring some "roommates" along and introduce them to him. Tell your roommates loud and clear where you are going and if they can pick you up at 10 o'clock.

Do not stay out longer than 10 o'clock in a strange city. That is asking for trouble, especially when you are in the company of someone you do not know.

Make an itinerary of the places to which you are going and leave them with trusted friends and family members. And stick to that itinerary. It is going to be very foolish if everybody thinks that you have gone off to see Chinatown and you decided to go off and see the local arts Museum. Who is going to know where you are in case something happens?

Driving Rules

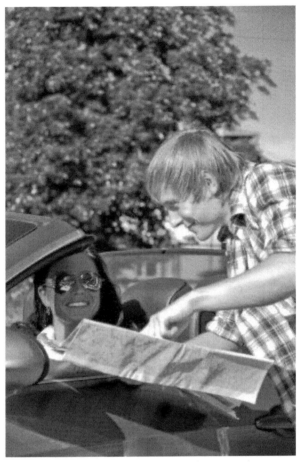

This is the road you take, fraulein!

If you are driving from one place to another, make sure that your vehicle is reliable. If you are renting it out, make sure that it is in excellent condition. You do not want to find yourself stranded 50 miles away from nowhere, with no chances of rescue in sight, do you?

Also, if you find yourself stranded, do not act like any foolish heroine in any stupid escapist novel, who writes "Going North" on the windscreen with her lipstick and moves off Southwest. That is so not funny. Also, you are not going to have a multibillionaire turning up to rescue you, because after all you are the heroine, all buxom, beautiful and brainless.

In reality, you may find yourself in circumstances beyond your control.

Abroad, there are plenty of travel clubs and AAA which can give you roadside assistance. Take full advantage of them. Make sure that your driving license is valid abroad. Also make sure that you have your country's embassy's number and address easily available.

Your baggage should be labeled properly with name, address and phone number. Use a luggage tag. Use your office number, work address and phone number on luggage tags in case your baggage gets lost. Do not leave this baggage unattended or under the responsibility of fellow passengers, while you go off to buy a cup of coffee in the lounge.

If you are driving, make sure you have not had one for the road at least 24 hours before driving. Have a good night's sleep before you set out. Have a full breakfast before you start to drive. Do not use electronic devices and cell phones while you are driving and definitely do not pick up any hitchhikers, even if they are women.

And never men, even if they look as innocent as turtledoves…

That sounds hard, but unfortunately it is a fact of life that men drivers were mugged by women hitchhikers, or their male accomplices who were hiding in the shadows somewhere. The moment a car stopped, the hitchhiker undulated up to the driver, cooed to him whether he could give her a lift to such and such place and during that time her partner in crime appeared to hold up the driver.

In the same way, if somebody offers to give you a ride, do not get taken for a ride. Smile politely, and say that you are waiting for your friend to pick you up. And then walk away and take out your cell phone.

Put it against your ear as if you are phoning, and if that person has stopped to see if someone really is coming to meet you, turn the cell phone towards him and face him. You may want to click his car number. Also, say it loud in his hearing. That should give him the idea that you are wide awake and you are transmitting his car information to somebody.

If he still persists on staying there, make a note of his car number on your cell phone and message it as well as your locality and the time to Pukar.

If you find yourself being held up in an ill lit area, give up your purse. After all, it does not have your important documents, and lots of money in it. In "Queen", Kangna did not give up her purse.[5] Instead, she kept shouting. No one came to her rescue. This is real life. She was not harmed, and beaten. This is escapist unreality. She could have been stabbed by the junkie.

But then she must had all her papers and credit cards in the purse, I presume.

If you are having any sort of problem with your car or vehicle, only accept help from authorized personnel and from the police.

Call AAA if alone and stranded.

---

[5] – Same movie trailer URL I posted about 12 pages above.

Travel Plans

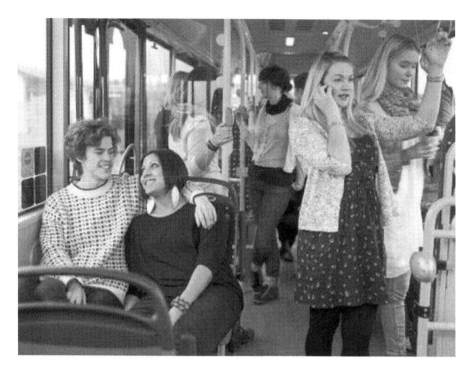

So, hello, Alison, I'll be there in 20 minutes. The pillar near the bridge you said? Hey, girl, you didn't ask that bore, Matt to join us did you? It's girls day out today. We'll go shopping, so get your credit cards along. I have some cash and my credit cards too. Ciao!

Do not tell all and sundry all about your travel plans. Consider your travel to someplace on a war footing. You are not broadcasting your strategy to the enemy, are you? And walls have ears.

And so, if you find yourself talking loudly in a public space about the places you are going to visit tomorrow, it is possible that some of the people surrounding you would want to visit that place tomorrow, and get within reach of you.

On the other hand, if you are talking on purpose, in order to mislead someone, well, go ahead. If he is of your own tourist group and has been a bit too persistent, you may want to tell other people of your tourist group that you intend to go to ABC place the next morning. And make sure your stalker sees you boarding a vehicle taking you to that particular place, the next morning.

Get off at the next stop and take the next transport to your real destination in itinerary. If he manages to catch the same vehicle you took, then look straight at him and start yelling. Tell everybody around you that you are being stalked. Make a fuss. Make a noise. Make him get off the vehicle. And then on to your original destination!

When you get back, tell everybody in your group what he did. You may want someone tougher than him to speak to him. Embarrass him. Tell the females around you in front of him to tell you immediately, if they saw him around you.

And if he still persists, you may want to spread the rumor that he is a stalker. You may also want to let your male tough acquaintances want to ask him what his intentions are. He is spoiling your holiday. Spoil his as far as you can.

Conclusion

So these are some commonsense safety tips, which can be utilized by women traveling solo.

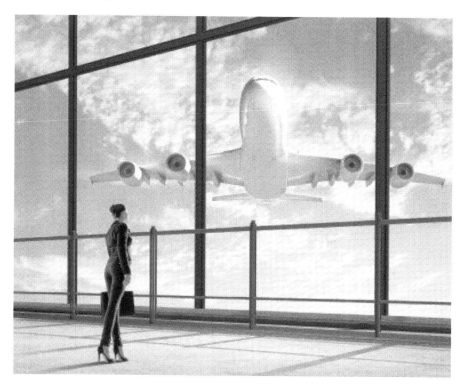

I am leaving on a jet plane, don't know when I'll be back again...

Remember to take out your health insurance with a reliable insurance company in your own country before you travel somewhere. Also, if you have medical insurance facilities, so much the better.

I asked a person who had traveled all over the world, how she managed to go off to strange places without worrying about finances. She said that she had enough of money in her account for a quick wire transfer. She also had people who knew where she was going. She kept in regular touch with them all through her trip.

So remember that there should be people who should know where you are, or at least have some knowledge about your general location.

Every country has its own travel and safety rules for women. So check them up, especially flight regulations and safety rules, before you catch your flight.

Reserve your place of stay beforehand. Confirm it, before you catch your flight. Make sure that you have another alternative destination where you could stay, in case of an emergency.

And always remember, what you think may not always come to pass. So if you go somewhere expecting to be confronted with horrors, it is better for you to stay home because you are in no state to travel anywhere. On the other hand, if you expect to enjoy your stay in a strange new world, you are going to find yourself enjoying yourself thoroughly.

So Spread Your Wings, and Fly. Fly Safe! Live Long and Prosper!

Author Bio

Dueep Jyot Singh is a Management and IT Professional who managed to gather Postgraduate qualifications in Management and English and Degrees in Science, French and Education while pursuing different enjoyable career options like being an hospital administrator, IT,SEO and HRD Database Manager/ trainer, movie , radio and TV scriptwriter, theatre artiste and public speaker, lecturer in French, Marketing and Advertising, ex-Editor of Hearts On Fire (now known as Solstice) Books Missouri USA, advice columnist and cartoonist, publisher and Aviation School trainer, ex-moderator on Medico.in, banker, student councilor ,travelogue writer … among other things!

One fine morning, she decided that she had enough of killing herself by Degrees and went back to her first love -- writing. It's more enjoyable! She already has 48 published academic and 14 fiction- in- different- genre books under her belt.

When she is not designing websites or making Graphic design illustrations for clients , she is browsing through old bookshops hunting for treasures, of which she has an enviable collection – including R.L. Stevenson, O.Henry, Dornford Yates, Maurice Walsh, De Maupassant, Victor Hugo, Sapper, C.N. Williamson, "Bartimeus" and the crown of her collection- Dickens "The Old Curiosity Shop," and so on… Just call her "Renaissance Woman") - collecting herbal remedies, acting like Universal Helping Hand/Agony Aunt, or escaping to her dear mountains for a bit of exploring, collecting herbs and plants and trekking.

Check out some of the other JD-Biz Publishing books

Gardening Series on Amazon

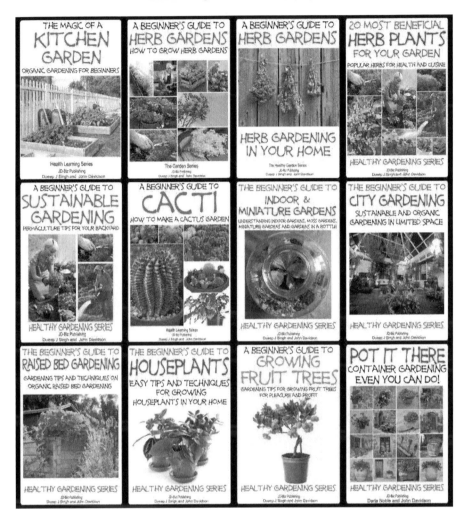

Health Learning Series

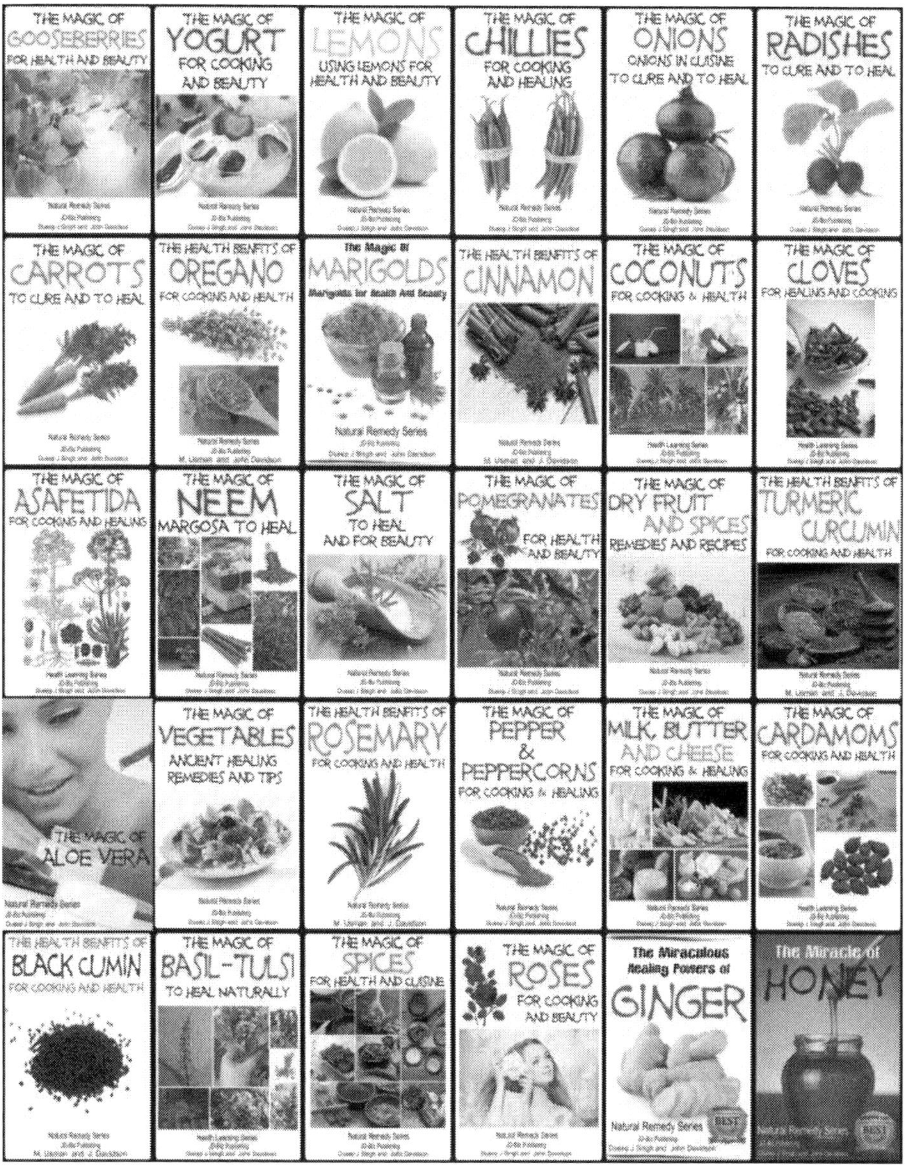

Country Life Books

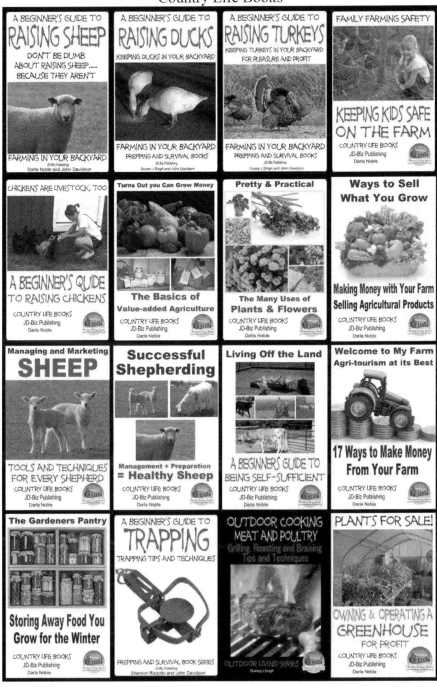

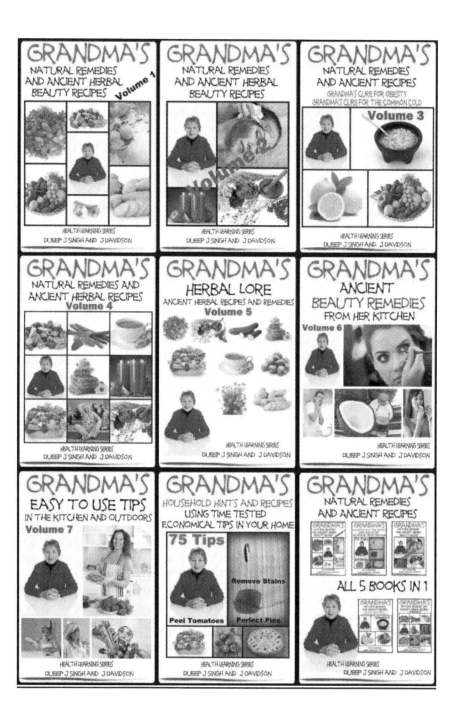

Health Learning Series

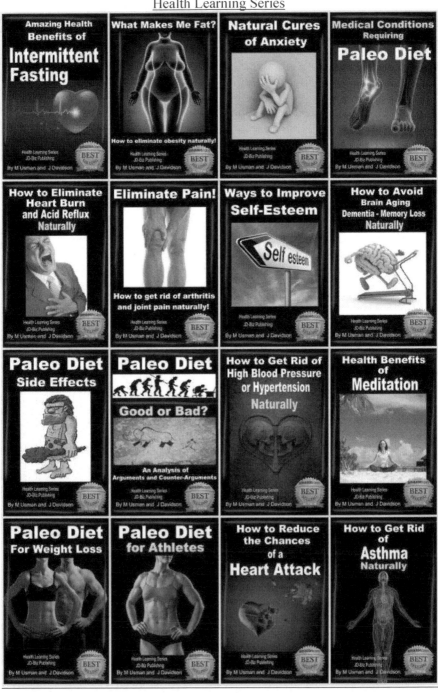

Amazing Animal Book Series

Learn To Draw Series

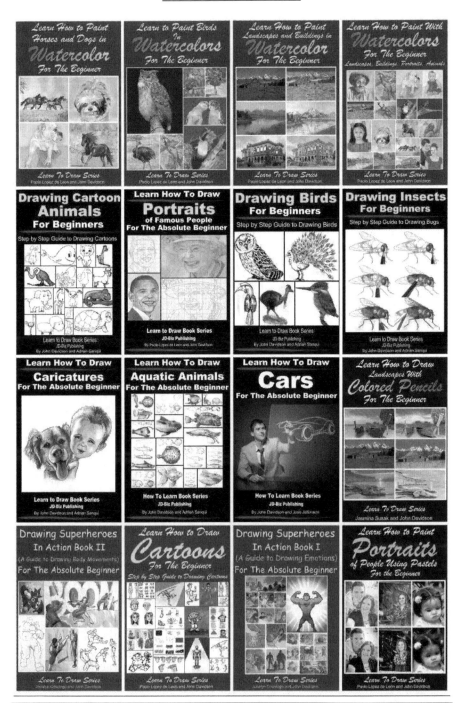

How to Build and Plan Books

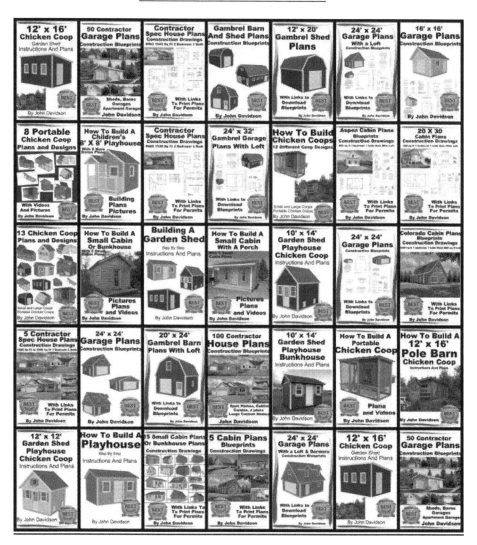

Entrepreneur Book Series

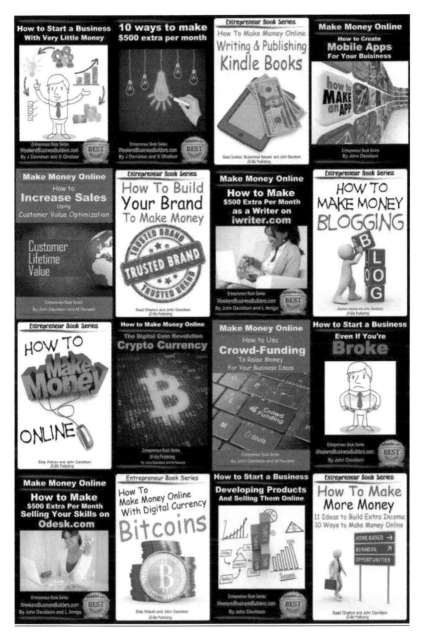

Our books are available at

1. Amazon.com
2. Barnes and Noble
3. Itunes
4. Kobo
5. Smashwords
6. Google Play Books

Publisher

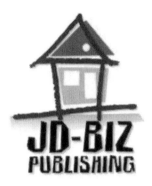

JD-Biz Corp

P O Box 374

Mendon, Utah 84325

http://www.jd-biz.com/

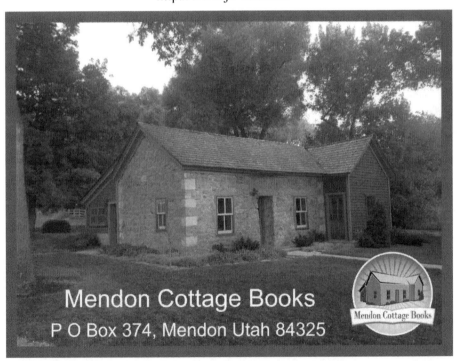